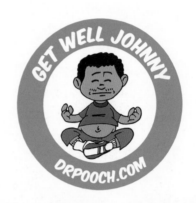

GET WELL JOHNNY
Book 4: He Stood Up For Himself!

By Dr. Pooch

Illustrations by Cuzzin' Dave

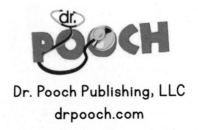

Dr. Pooch Publishing, LLC
drpooch.com

Get Well Johnny
Book 4: He Stood Up For Himself!
Copyright © 2015 by Dr. Pooch
Published by Dr. Pooch Publishing, LLC

ISBN: 978-0-9964667-0-7

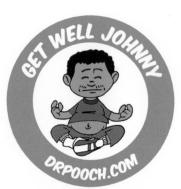

The Dr. Pooch Foundation

The Dr. Pooch Foundation is a nonprofit 501(c)(3) organization whose mission is to create and implement holistic health curriculum for schools and communities across the world. To change our world, we must begin with ourselves. Dr. Pooch Foundation programs increase and cultivate health and wellness awareness and nurture holistic health literacy. We are all connected to the whole. Let's learn new healthy ways and unlearn old destructive habits together to make a better more sustainable world for us ALL!

Donations and contributions to the Dr. Pooch Foundation go a long way towards increasing resources to ensure every child is not only health-literate, but holistic health-literate! Scan this QR Code to DONATE!

For more info: visit **drpooch.com**

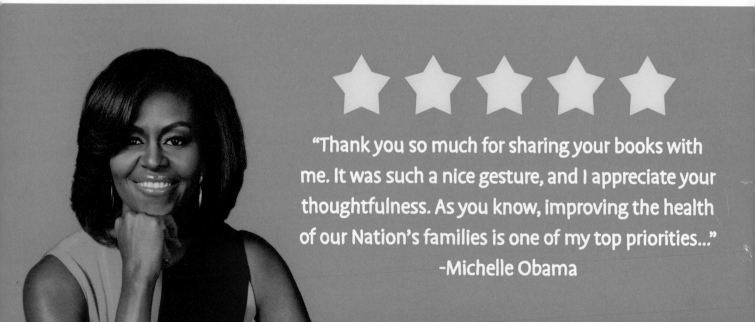

"Thank you so much for sharing your books with me. It was such a nice gesture, and I appreciate your thoughtfulness. As you know, improving the health of our Nation's families is one of my top priorities..."
-Michelle Obama

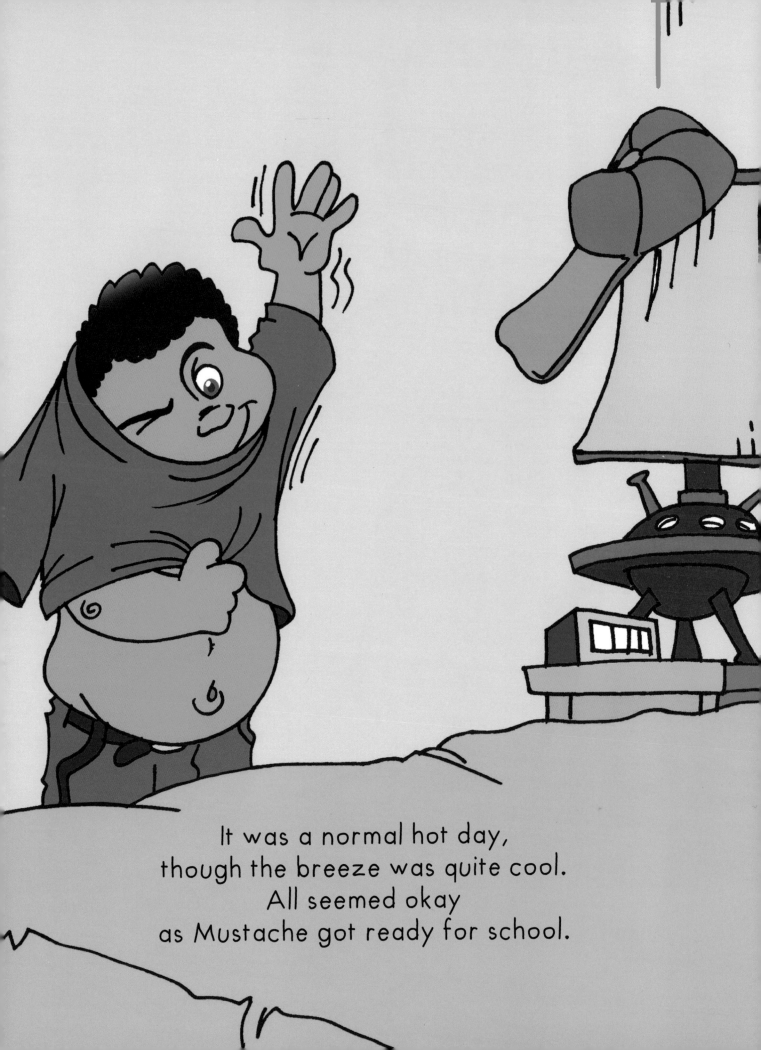

It was a normal hot day,
though the breeze was quite cool.
All seemed okay
as Mustache got ready for school.

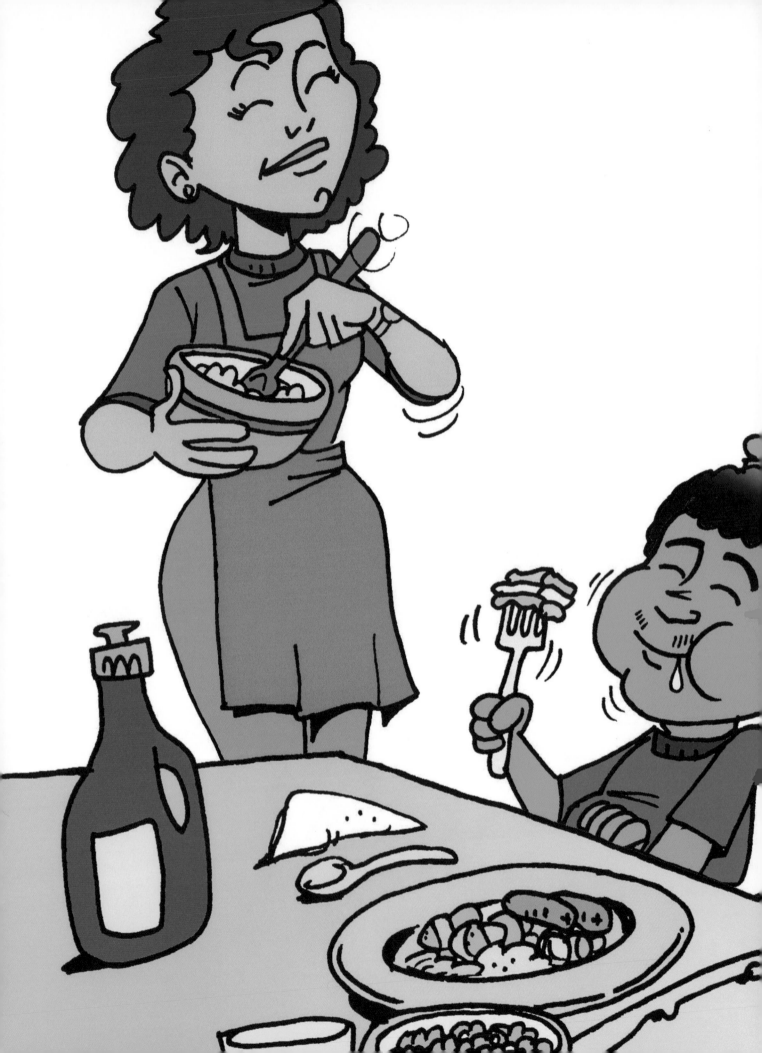

He had a wholesome breakfast
that Mom made from scratch.
Pancakes from whole flour,
he ate the whole batch!

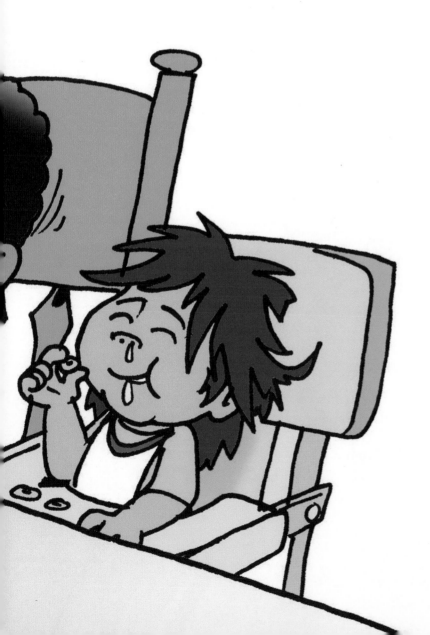

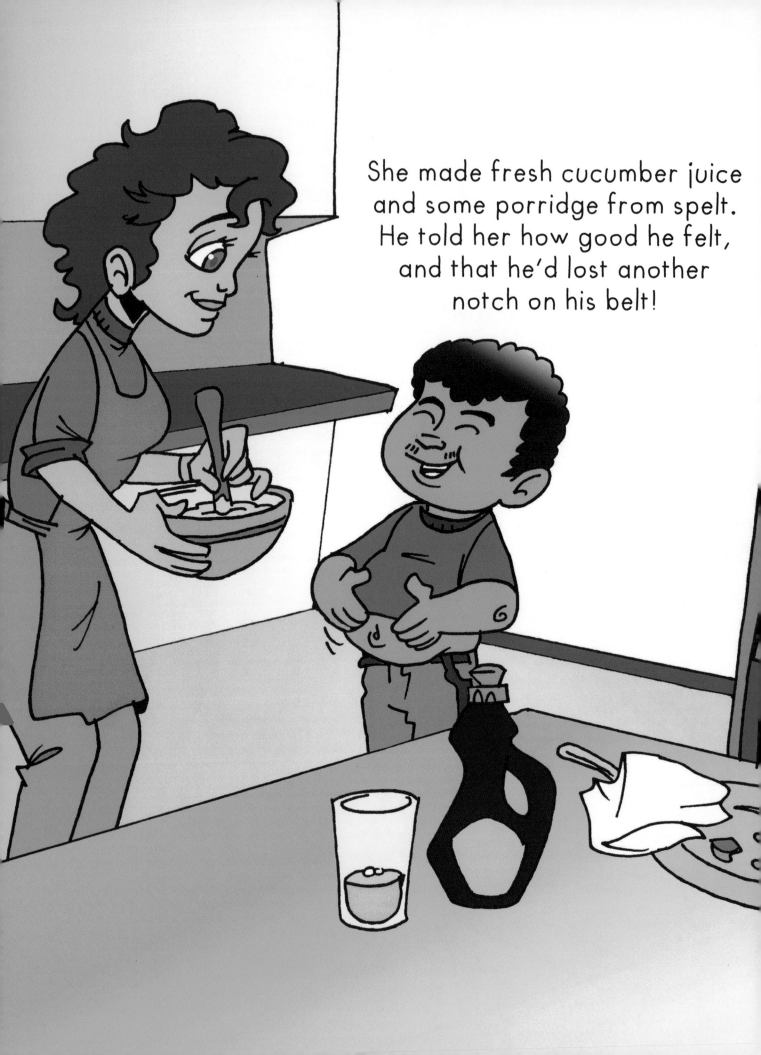

She made fresh cucumber juice
and some porridge from spelt.
He told her how good he felt,
and that he'd lost another
notch on his belt!

She said, "It's because of all the good foods you eat.
Whole grain cereals, whole fruits and clean meats."

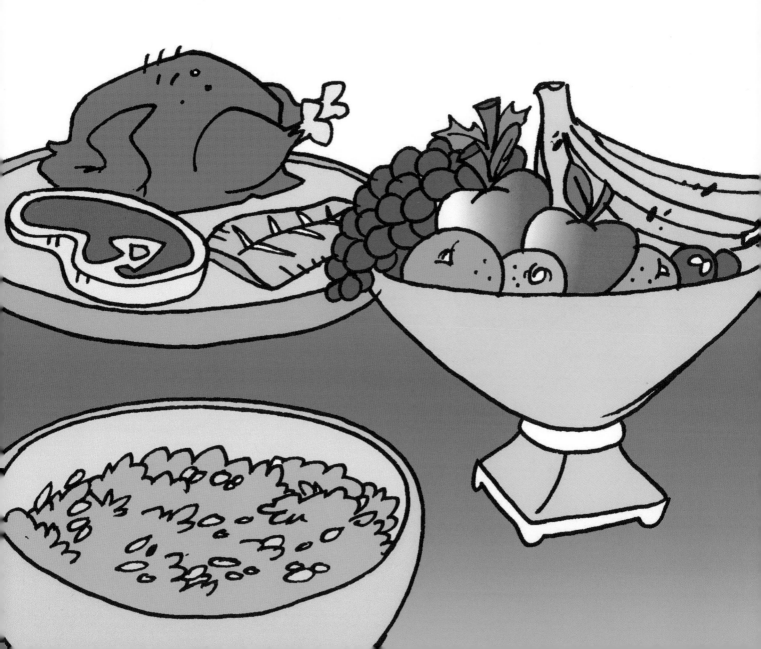

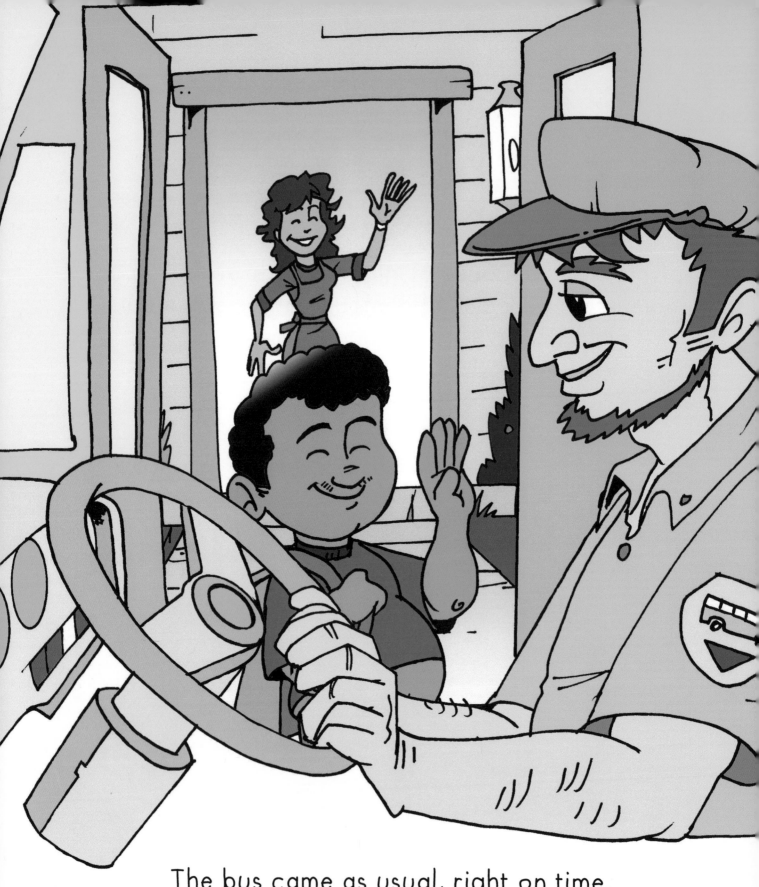

The bus came as usual, right on time.
"How are you, Mr. Bus Driver?"
The bus driver said, "Fine."

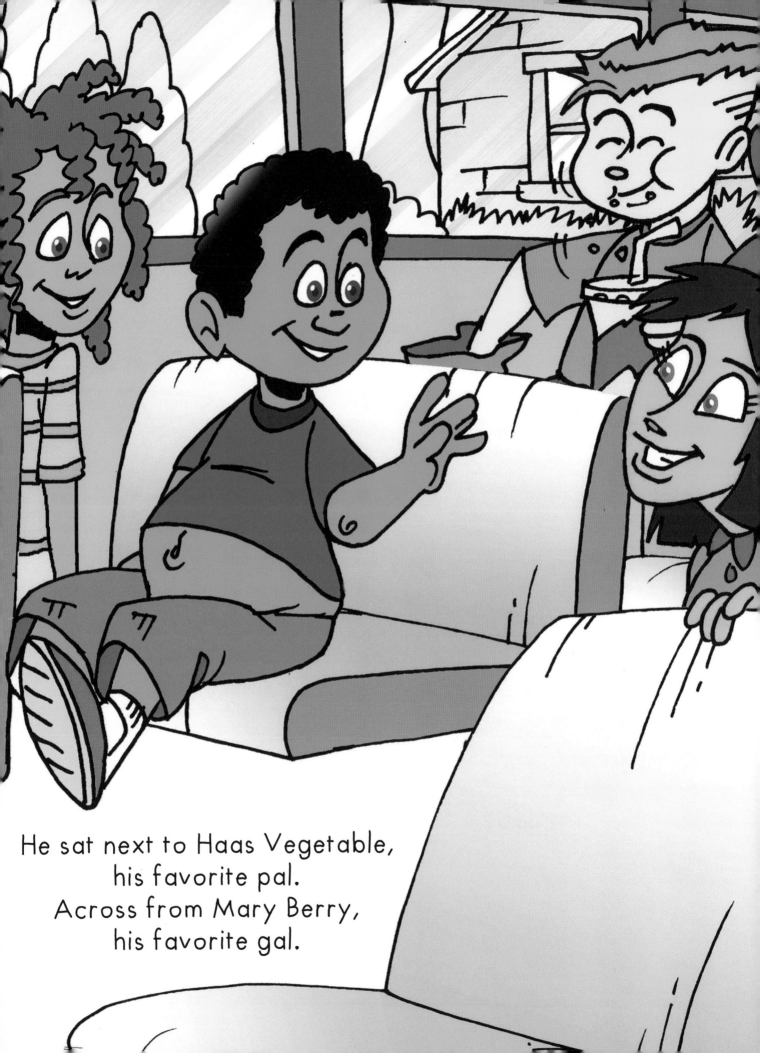

He sat next to Haas Vegetable,
his favorite pal.
Across from Mary Berry,
his favorite gal.

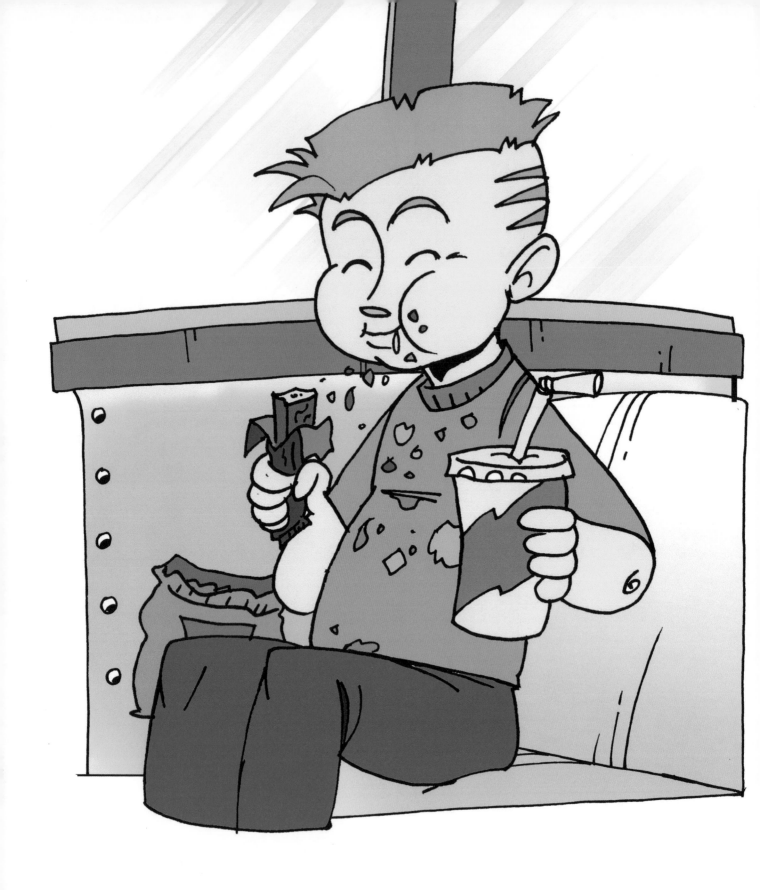

Petey Peachfuzz was sitting in the back,
making loud noises and eating sugary snacks.

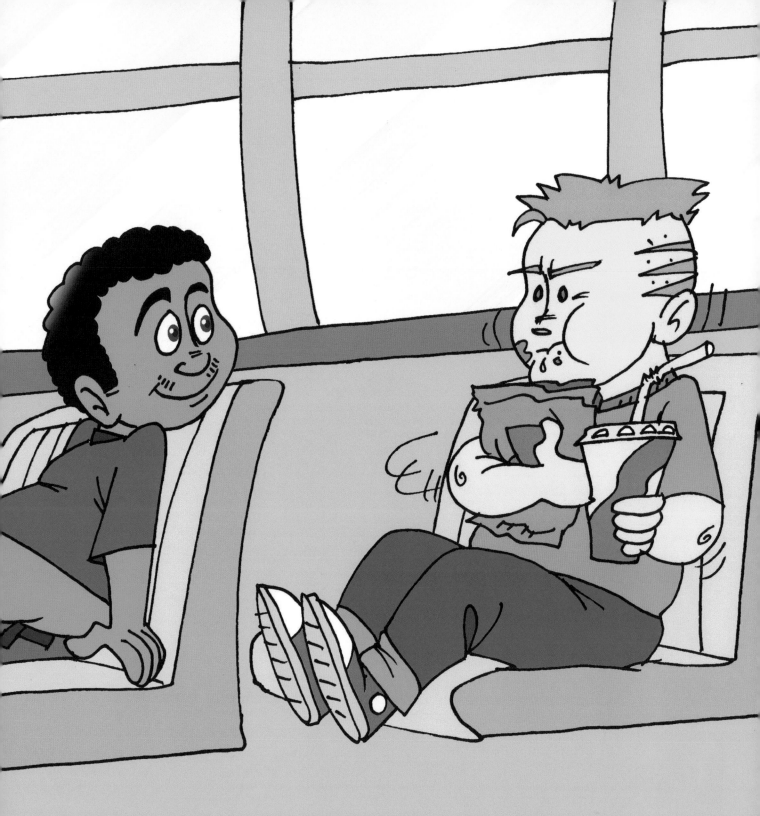

Johnny Mustache looked at Petey Peachfuzz
and Petey looked back, saying,
"I'm not giving you any of my snacks.
And, besides, you're too fat!"

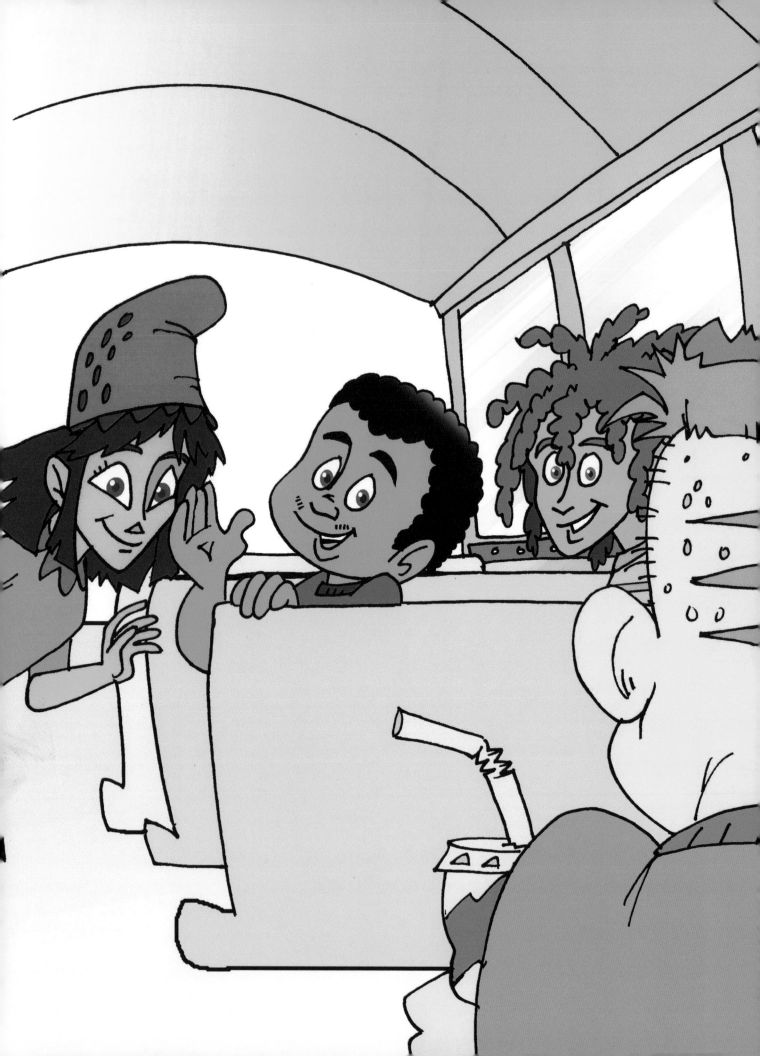

Mustache surprised, replied,
"I am who I am, but I'm surely not your friend.
And you're not mine,
because my friends are kind."

Mary Berry and Haas Vegetable said,
"Don't worry, Johnny, you're not fat,
you just have a big body!"

They all laughed about it as they pulled up to school.
They rushed off to class and followed all rules.

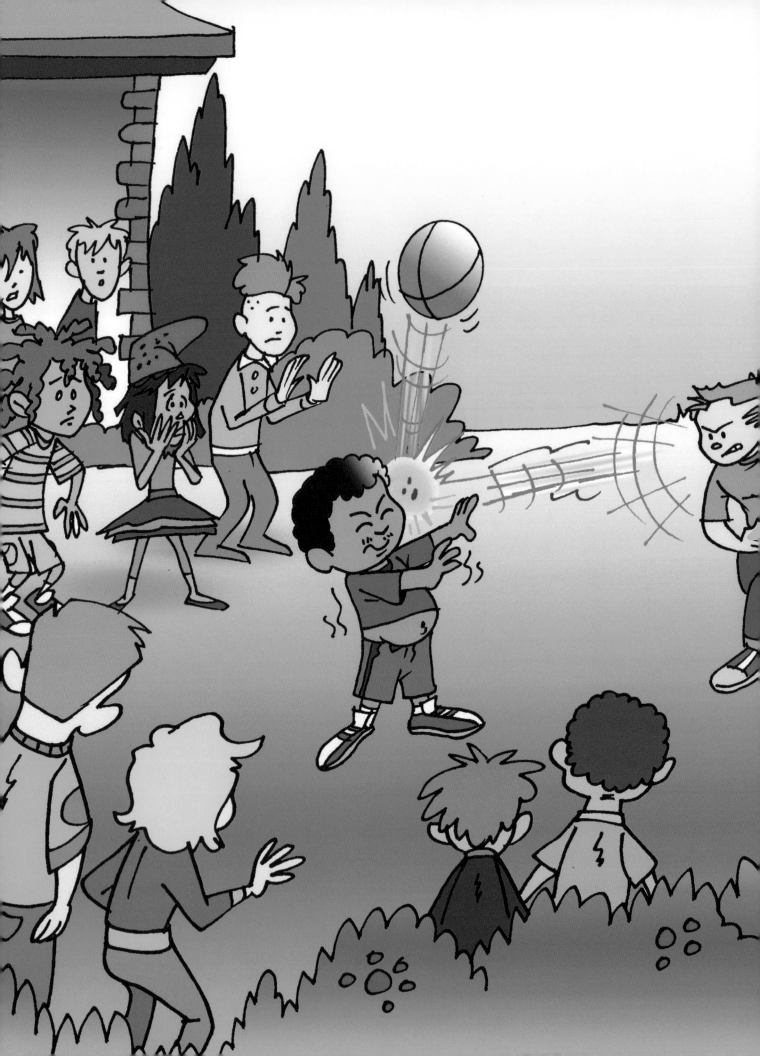

At recess they played games,
like freeze tag and chase.
Until Petey Peachfuzz threw a ball
at Mustache's face!

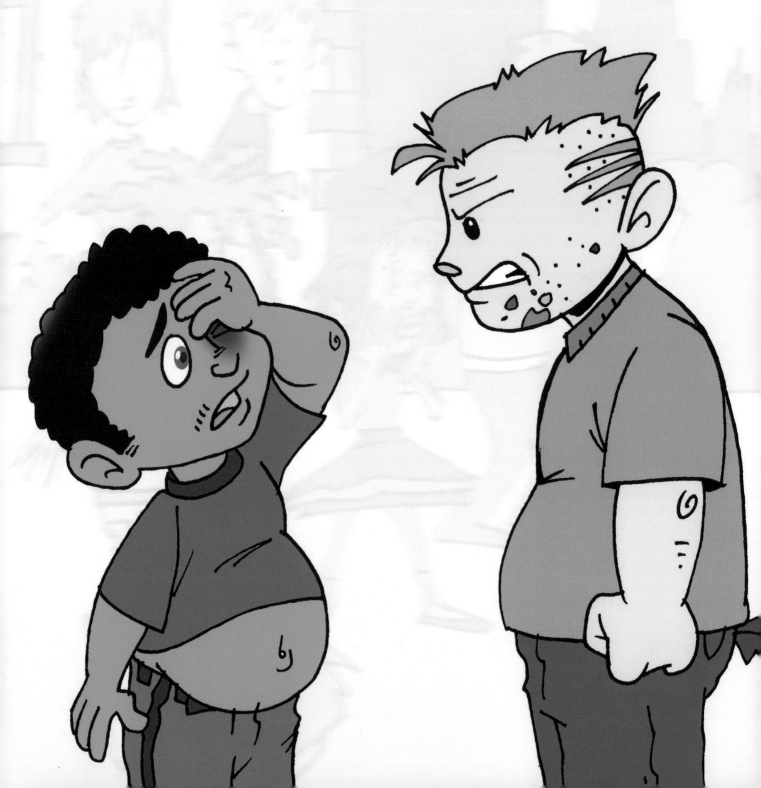

Everyone on the playground said,
"Go away, Petey Peachfuzz, you don't play nice."

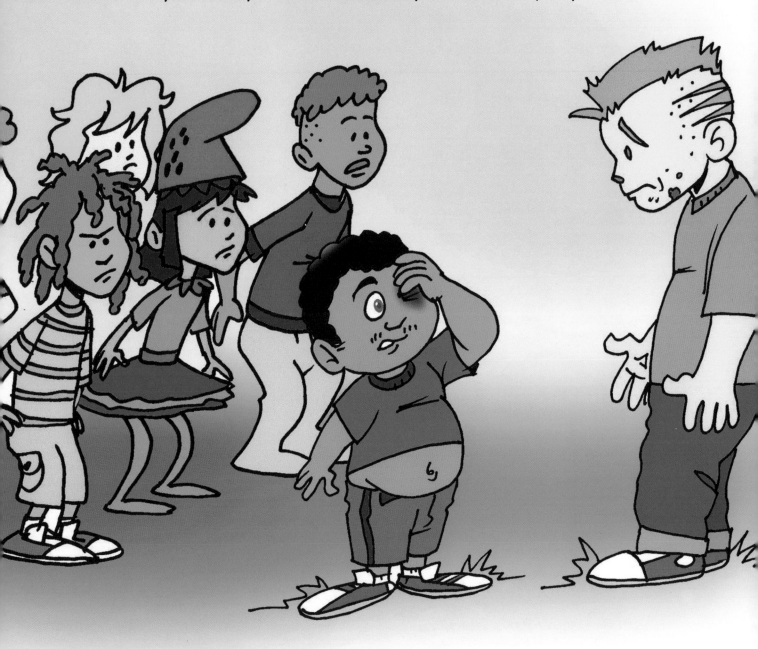

"We'll all tell the teacher and you'll pay the price!"

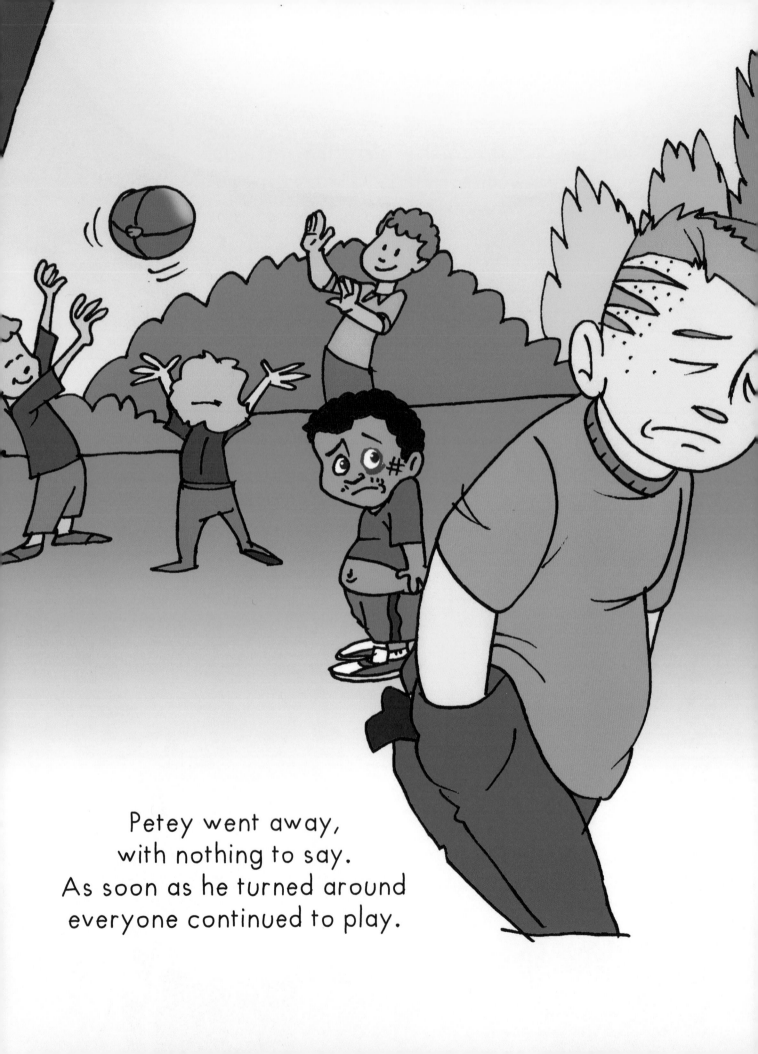

Petey went away,
with nothing to say.
As soon as he turned around
everyone continued to play.

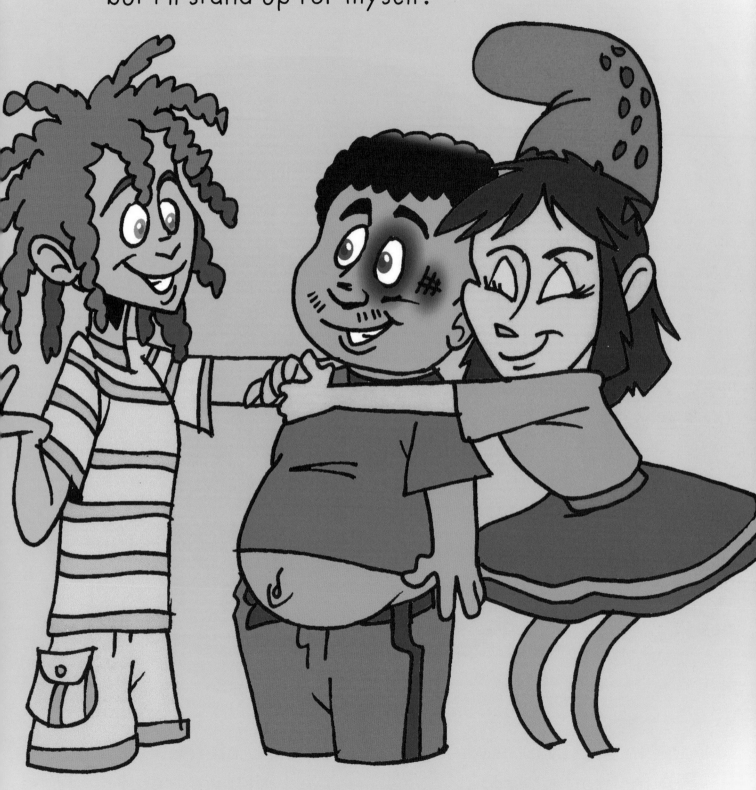

Mustache said, "Thanks, guys, but I'll stand up for myself."

They replied, "We know that, Johnny, but we're here to help!"

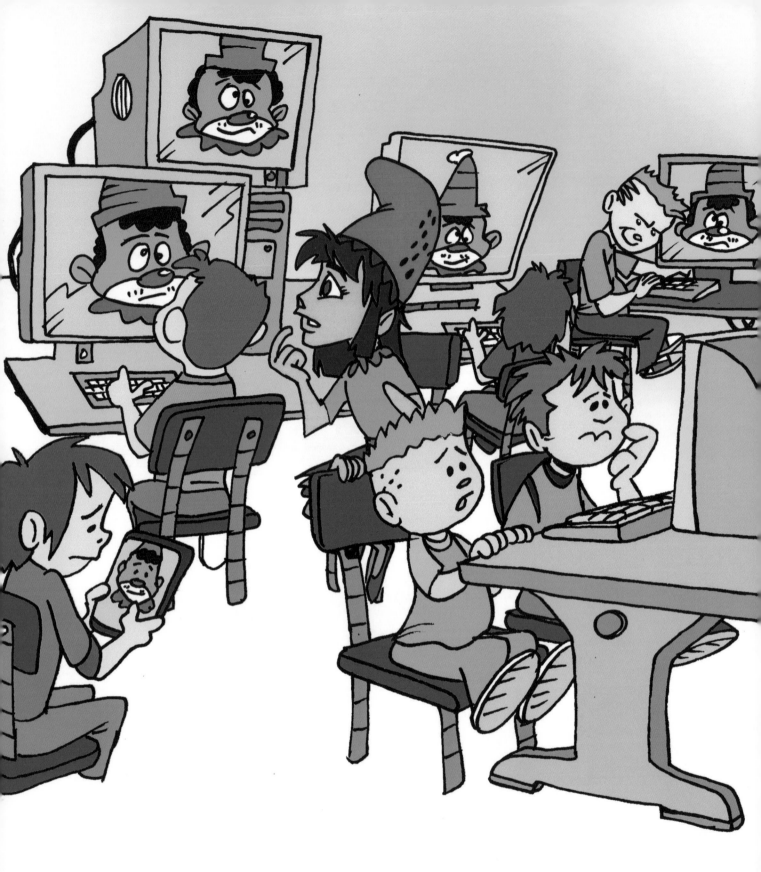

Back in class, everyone began to work on their computers.
But instead of working, Petey used his to spread rumors!

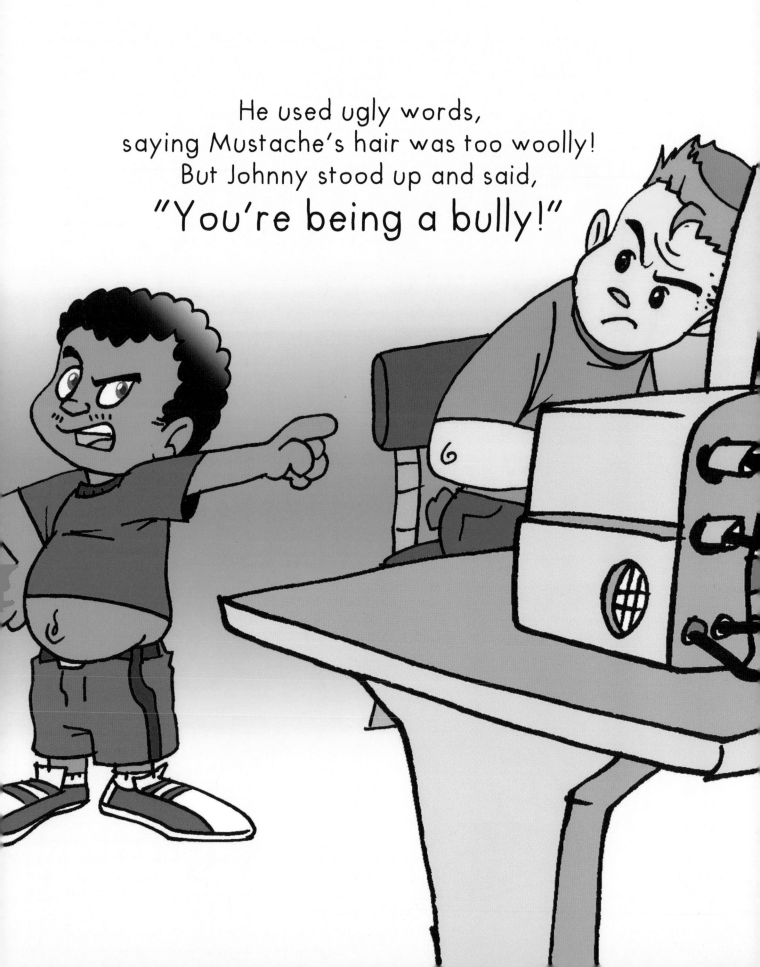

He used ugly words,
saying Mustache's hair was too woolly!
But Johnny stood up and said,
"You're being a bully!"

"I might be overweight, but I'm changing what I eat.
Unlike you, always eating bad sugars and sweets!"

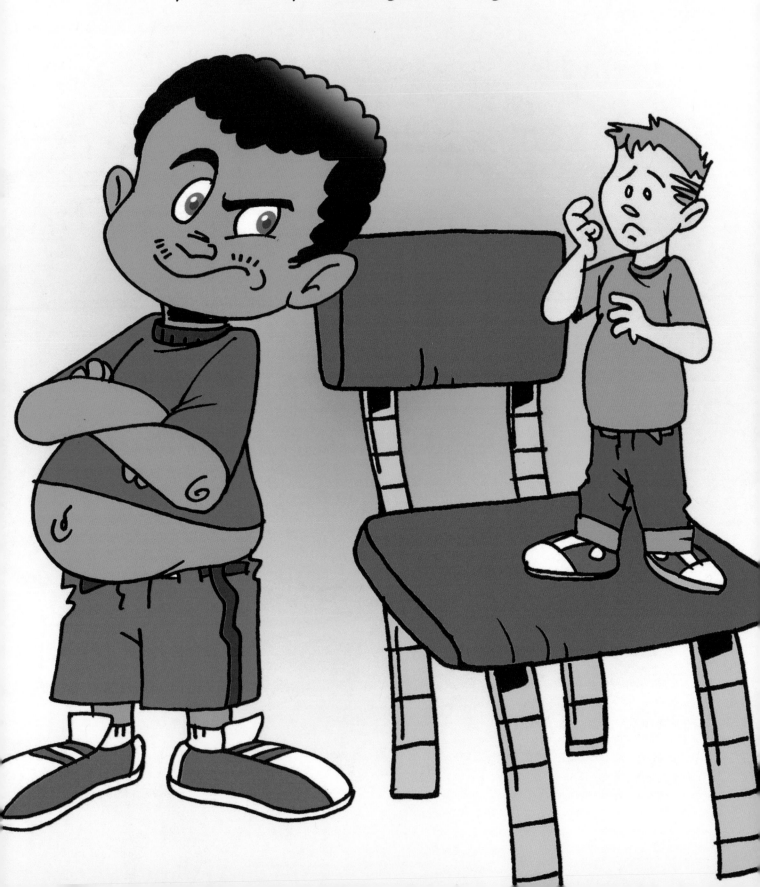

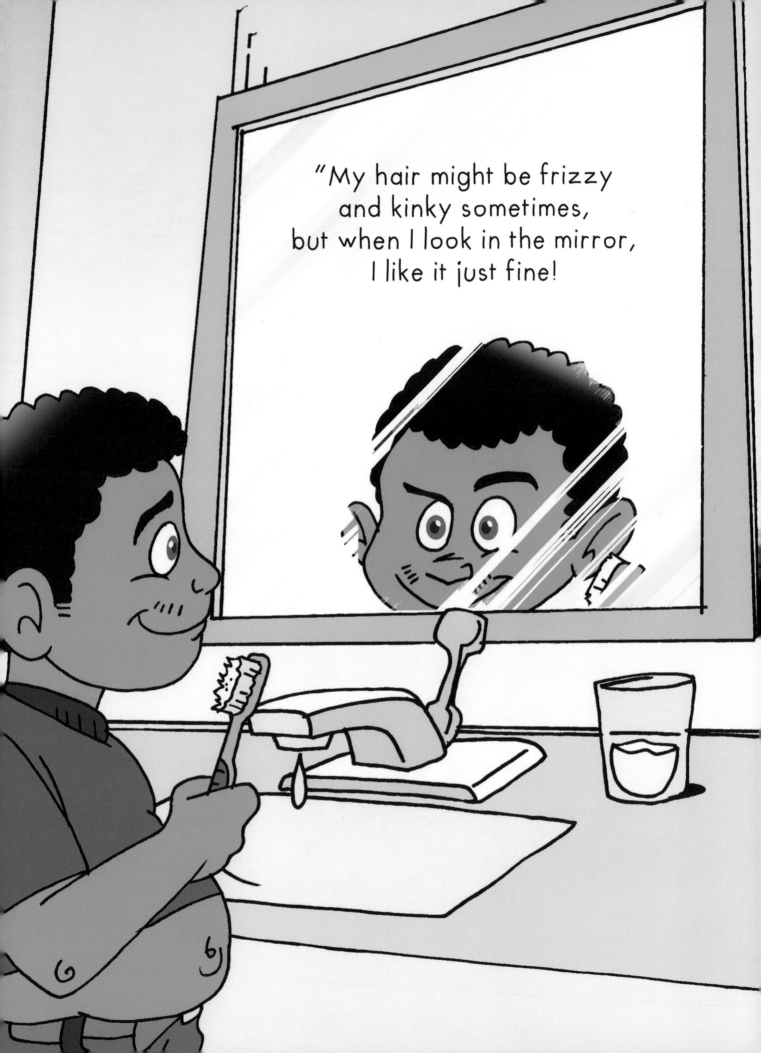

My shoes aren't name brand
and my clothes are a bit worn.
Because there were no silver
spoons where I was born!

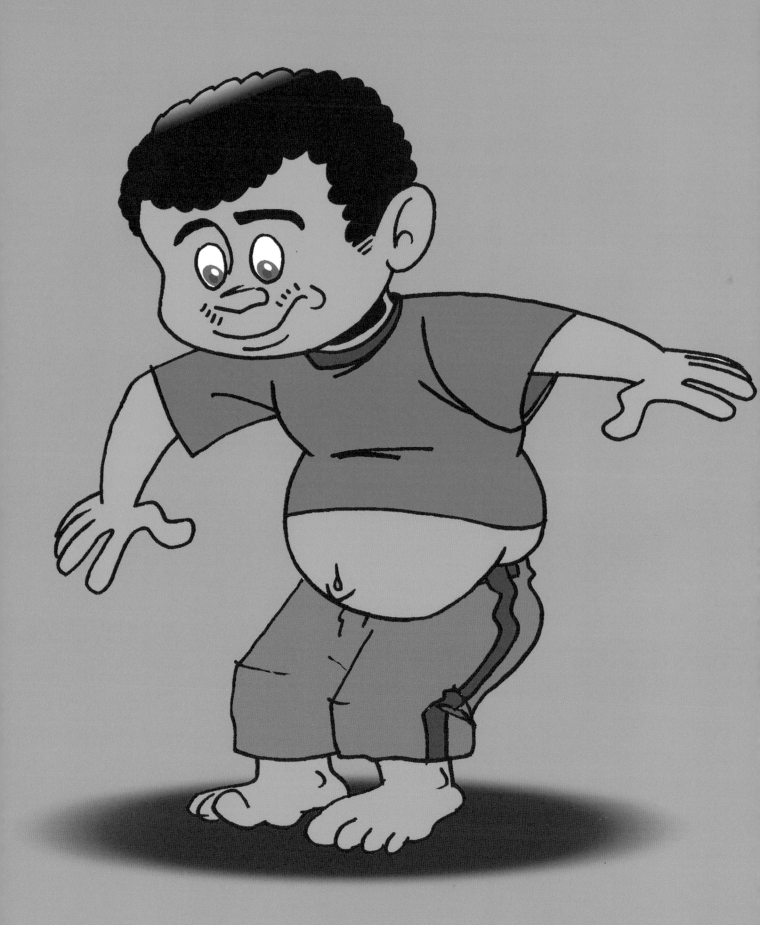

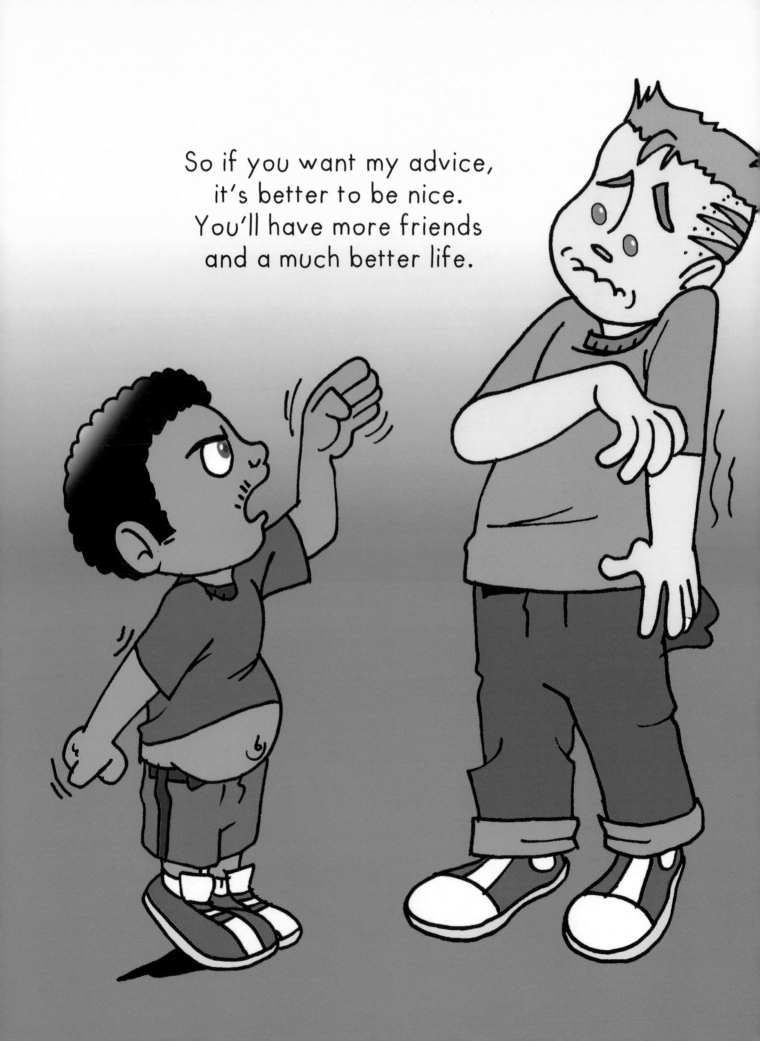

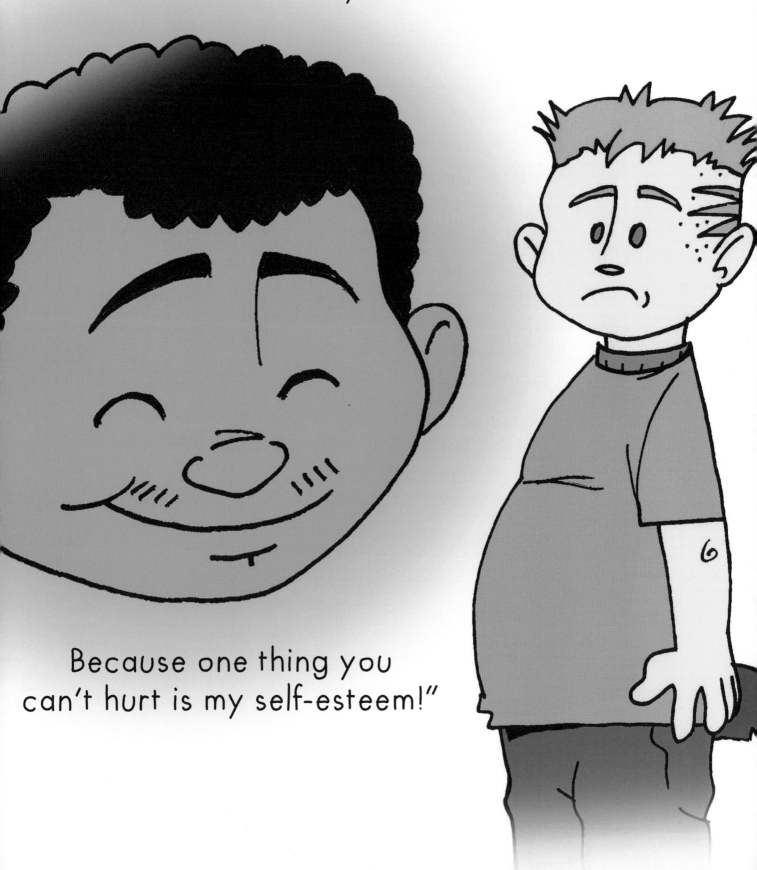

But it doesn't harm me
if you choose to be mean.

Because one thing you
can't hurt is my self-esteem!"

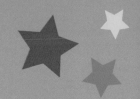

AFFIRMATIONS

Underline the important word in each sentence.

1. I am happy.
2. I am healthy.
3. I am smart.
4. I am funny.
5. I am strong.
6. I am loved.

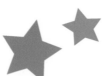

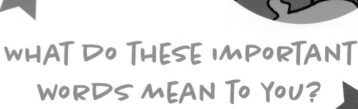

WHAT DO THESE IMPORTANT WORDS MEAN TO YOU?

Now, write a sentence about each of the underlined words.

1. _____

2. _____

3. _____

4. _____

5. _____

6. _____

REMEMBER: The important words to remember about yourself are HAPPY, HEALTHY, SMART, FUNNY, STRONG, LOVED.

TAKING YOUR POWER BACK

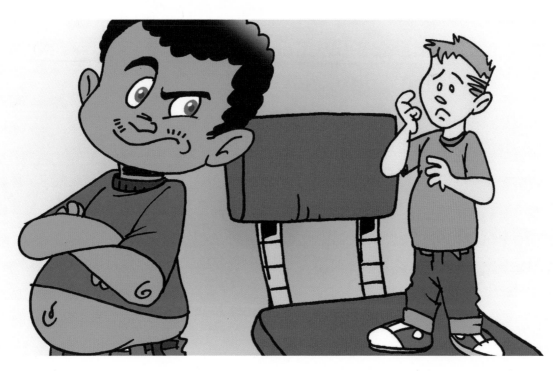

Being bullied or not being your highest Self makes you feel small. Remembering your true and highest Self gives you your power back!

Tell the world, in a few sentences, who You truly are and who You want to Become!

_____

_____

_____

_____

_____

_____

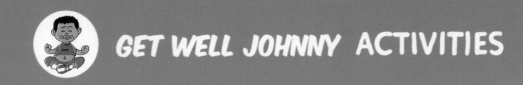
IN SOMEONE ELSE'S SHOES

Bullying another person (hurting them or their feelings) also causes harm to the perpetrator. Jealousy and anger harm the heart of those who hold those feelings.

What do you think Petey Peachfuzz is thinking in this illustration?

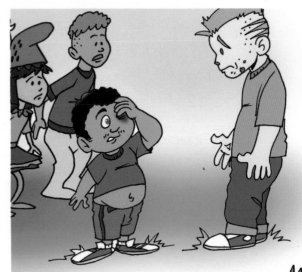

FINDING EMPATHY

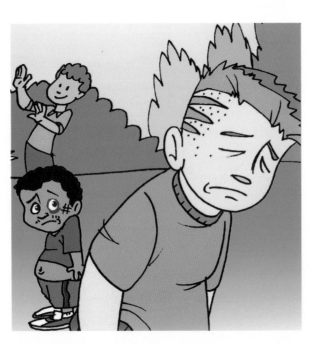

To find love in your heart for someone who's hurt you is difficult but necessary to heal from the trauma. Hatred and resentment harm the heart of those who hold them inside.

What do you think Get Well Johnny is thinking in this illustration?

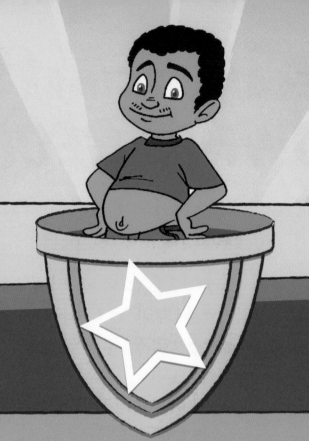

ANTI-BULLYING CONTRACT

I, _____ , will not allow anyone to hurt me.
       YOUR NAME

I, _____ , will not hurt others.
       YOUR NAME

I, _____ , will stand up for myself
       YOUR NAME

I, _____ , will stand up for others.
       YOUR NAME

I, _____ , will ask an adult if I need help.
       YOUR NAME

This contract was written on the _____ day of the month
of_____in the year_____ , and is a
binding contract between Dr. Pooch and myself.

_____
          YOUR SIGNATURE

This contract is not legally binding but is to be signed as a commitment against bullying.

REGGIE REGIMEN'S
BROWNIE RECIPE

Hi, my name is Reggie Regimen and together we'll make fun, great tasting raw recipes!

WHAT YOU'LL NEED IS:

- 4 Cups **Walnuts**
- 5 Cups **Dates**
- 2 Cups **Raw Cacao Powder**
- ½ Teaspoon **Sea Salt**

INSTRUCTIONS:

(With the help of an adult)

1. Put all ingredients into a food processor little by little while mixing.
2. Place in a pan. Spread out.
3. Cut out into squares.

And voila! Ready to eat raw brownies. No cooking necessary!

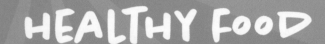

HEALTHY FOOD

Eating raw foods like fresh, organic fruits, vegetables, seeds, and nuts make you strong, healthy, and smart!

COLOR ME!

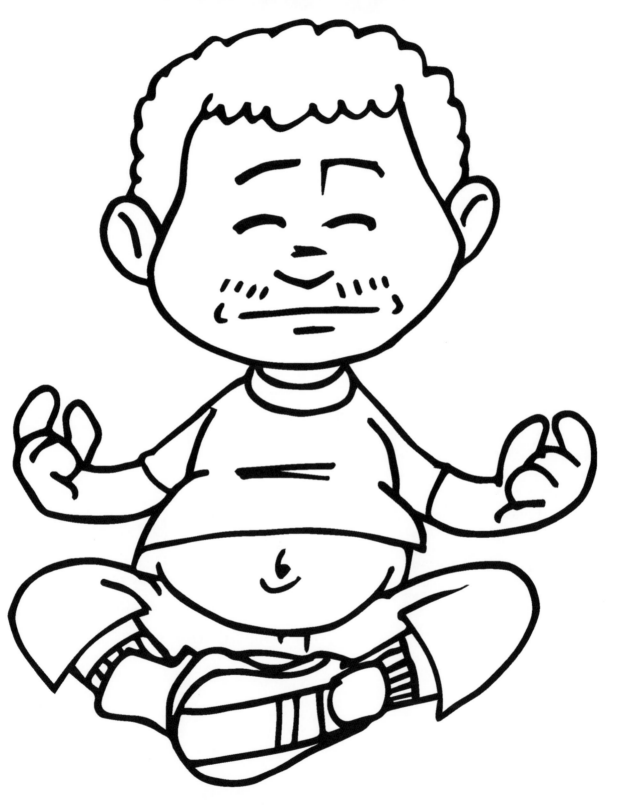

GET WELL JOHNNY

WEEKLY CHECKLIST

This Activity Sheet Belongs To: _____

✔ **Instructions:** Place a checkmark on each thing you've done each day this week!

This is a weekly checklist kids and/or parents can use to gage where they are in the application of each book's learnings. *Photocopy as needed.*	Sunday	Monday	Tuesday	Wednesday	Thursday	Friday	Saturday
Did I help someone today? *Being of service to someone is the ultimate gift.*							
Did anyone bully me today? *Find someone you trust and tell them what happened. No one should be bullied.*							
Am I happy today? *Happiness is a cornerstone in maintaining good health.*							
Am I worried about anything? *Stress and anxiety are growing topics, let's talk about it.*							
Did I laugh really hard today? *Besides walking, laughing is one our best medicines!*							
Did I poo poo today? *#2 is serious business. Chronic constipation can lead to many health problems. Poop everyday!*							

HEALTHY CHOICES: Why are healthy habits important? Take notes!

_____

_____

_____

Find fun activities at the end of all Get Well Johnny Books and visit **www.drpooch.com** to learn more!

He Stood Up For Himself!
Book 4

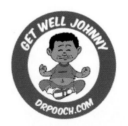

Printed in Great Britain
by Amazon